The Don't Panic Guide to Birth

2nd Edition

Ask a Midwife Series: Book Two

Fiona McArthur

Illustrated by Bettina Dwyer

First published 2009
Text copyright © Fiona McArthur 2015.
Revised second edition 2016

ISBN-13:

978-1532912917

ISBN-10:

1532912919

About the author 1

Is this labour? 5

I want my baby now! 13

Can I bring on labour? 17

Will I be safe at home in early labour? ..25

What if my waters haven't broken? 31

What's the secret to breathing? 35

Hospital and settling in 41

Checking on baby 49

What if my labour needs to be induced? 51

Drugs and pain relief 61

The stages of labour 69

The first hour after birth 79

Breastfeeding 93

Making the most of your hospital stay 95

Your birth plan 99

Your hospital bag 105

A quick word on the unexpected 111

Acknowledgments...113

About the author

Fiona McArthur is a Registered Nurse/Practising Clinical Nurse Specialist in Midwifery, with over twenty-five years' experience as a midwife. She is passionate about parent education and birth classes, and, for the last eight years, has also been involved with obstetric emergency education for midwives and doctors. She is a multi-published fiction and non-fiction author and is married with five sons. Fiona lives in regional New South Wales.

.

INTRODUCTION

You're almost there. You've reached the final few weeks of pregnancy, and you're about to come face-to-face with this new little person in your life. Now all that stands between the two of you is . . . birth.

This book is designed to answer all those last-minute questions that you, and those sharing your birth experience with you, might have. As a midwife, I'm privileged to meet brand-new babies every day of my working life.

But this is your baby, your birth, and your personal miracle.

The birth of your baby will be an amazing, exhausting, incredible experience. Some mothers will push out their baby with surprising ease and others won't find it quite so easy. Others may finish with an unexpected caesarean birth.

The aim of this book is to outline the choices available and to give you the information you need to make those choices. Every single birth is different and unpredictable – that's part of the wonder of childbirth. But knowing what might happen, and what options you have, can help make your birth experience positive. The one thing you can be certain of is that the birth of your baby will be worth the effort.

When you're approaching birth, fear is the worst companion you can have. The good news is that you can control fear with knowledge. In this book, I've drawn on information from my professional friends, my experience as both a midwife and a mother of five sons, and from the answers to questions asked by great couples and fabulous young mums in antenatal classes.

By the way, throughout this book you'll notice that I've called your baby 'she' ('she/ he' is too impersonal for me). If you think or have been told that you're having a boy, just substitute 'he'. (You never can be sure until right at the end, when you see all the 'bits', anyway!) Similarly, I've talked of doctors and midwives as 'she'. Sorry, guys.

So, let's talk about the birth of your baby.

Each chapter will take you about five minutes to read..

1

Is this labour?

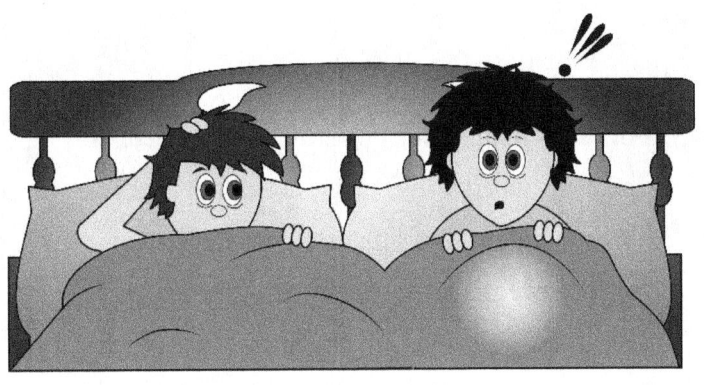

So, what happens when you go into labour? How does it work and how do you know it's the real thing?

At full-term (forty weeks, or two hundred and forty days, from the first day of your last period), your uterus or womb is about the size of a watermelon, with a thick and closed circular opening at the bottom called the cervix. The cervix is a muscle that stays closed during pregnancy to keep the baby supported within the womb.

In order to open for birth, the cervix needs to be softened by a hormone called prostaglandin that's naturally produced at the end of pregnancy. Also, a pattern of regular contractions needs to be established by the muscles embedded in the uterus, to pull the cervix up so that the bottom of the uterus is thin and ready to open.

There are various signs that labour is beginning – you are likely to experience some or all of these:

- As the end of your pregnancy draws near, the cervical canal or narrow opening at the bottom of your uterus (where the sperm entered all those months ago) softens and opens a little, allowing the mucous plug that sealed the canal from the outside world to fall away. Some people call this plug the 'show'. You probably won't notice that the show has fallen out until you go to the toilet and wipe yourself. This could happen as you start labour contractions or as early as three weeks before, so don't rush to the hospital if you see a lump of mucus, possibly with a smear of blood, on the toilet tissue; just ring up the maternity ward or your midwife for advice.

- Another sign of labour is that the bag of waters that your baby is floating in breaks or springs a leak. (Despite what you hear, only around one in ten women's waters break before they begin contractions.) If that happens, you might feel a strange pop-like sensation, or suddenly find that your underwear is wet. The fluid (called amniotic fluid) will keep dribbling and you won't be able to control it. If you put a pad on, you'll be able to see how much fluid is coming out. It's common for women towards the end of pregnancy to have an increase in vaginal mucus, so damp underwear might not be a sign of broken waters. But if you need to change a soaked pad your waters have probably broken, and the fluid will usually keep dripping in fits and starts until your baby is born.

Once your waters have broken, the uterine environment is no longer sealed and there's a greater chance of infection making its way through to your baby, so call the hospital and ask for their advice on safety issues. Your caregiver (midwife or doctor) needs to know what time your waters break – make a mental note or get your birth partner to write it down – in order to keep an eye out for infection.

The colour of the amniotic fluid draining from around the baby is important. It should be clear like tap water, or slightly pink with flecks of white (little globs of vernix, a skin-protecting substance coating the baby that disappears as you approach your due date). The colour of amniotic fluid gives us a clue on how baby is travelling. That's why it's good to talk to your caregiver when your water breaks. If you develop a fever (temperature), go straight in to hospital or see your caregiver to have a check.

If your amniotic fluid is green, brown, red or bright yellow, visit your nearest maternity ward, as this can be an indication of infection or stress on baby. If you develop a fever (temperature), go straight in to hospital.

- You may not notice the show and your waters may not break. The first sign that your labour is beginning might be the onset of contractions.

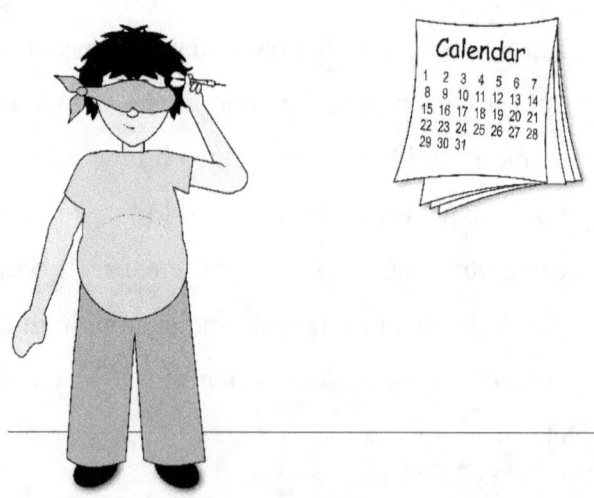

At first, when the cervix is just beginning to soften, the contractions are often painless, or at least much less painful than the true contractions of labour. Braxton Hicks contractions mostly feel like tightness in your abdomen, as if the baby is pushing against your belly or chest. Sometimes, they might feel like period pain, either in the back or in the front where bikini pants would sit. These 'practice' contractions, which help to prepare your body for birth, are usually infrequent, do not last long and do not continue to get stronger and closer together (unlike true labour contractions). They may be regular for a time, but speed up and slow down. Go with the flow and let them happen, as it may take a couple of days, a week or even more for your body to be ready. One way to tell whether your body is just practising is to change your physical activity (walk around if you've been sitting down, or vice versa) and see what the contractions do. Practice contractions often go away with a change of activity, meaning that you are not in full labour yet.

- True labour starts when you feel regular, wave-like contractions that are painful. Think of waves at the beach; you ride up the front of the wave until the height of the contraction, then back down the wave as the contraction recedes.

> '*My belly felt like a board every fifteen minutes and then the cramps started to hurt. I'd had a few false starts so didn't tell anyone for a while.*'
>
> **Vicki, 32 years,**
>
> **first-time mum**

2

I want my baby now!

Don't be surprised if you begin to feel impatient as you approach your baby's due date. You're fed up, you're uncomfortable and you want your baby NOW. Why can't the doctor bring on your labour?

Just remember that your baby will come when she's ready. So, as long as you and your baby are well and your waters haven't broken, don't waste energy wishing it would happen. These are your final moments with your baby inside. Hug her to yourself – just the two of you in secret communication.

Be selfish at this special time. Relax, chill out and enjoy it. This last secret time between you and your baby is precious beyond words.

Labour happens when the hormones in your body decide that it's time to birth your baby. It doesn't necessarily happen on your due date , or when your mother can come to stay, or when you expect it.

Officially, labour is expected to occur forty weeks after the first day of your last period. In reality, you can expect to labour naturally sometime over a four-week period: from two weeks before your due date to two weeks after. If you go into labour earlier than thirty-seven weeks, your labour is 'premature', and your doctor and midwives will need to take special steps to prepare for an early birth. If you haven't gone into labour by forty-two weeks, you are 'overdue'; your doctor will discuss induction with you as this date approaches.

Babies are often late. Your pregnancy may feel like the longest in history, but it's not. The recommended time for a doctor to intervene is after your baby is ten days past your Estimated Date of Confinement or Birth (the 'EDC' or 'EDB' on your antenatal card).

At this stage of your pregnancy, ten days can seem like an eternity! But if you think about it, you'll realise that this extra waiting isn't so bad. Statistics show that if you have an induction (that is, try to bring on labour with drugs or by breaking your waters), you increase your risk of more intervention: medicated pain relief, epidural, forceps or vacuum extractions. The ultimate intervention is a caesarean section, which increases the chance of your baby needing to be admitted to a special-care nursery, as well as the chance of your next baby being born by caesarean.

So, although it's hard to be patient and wait that extra week when you've already waited so many, you can see why it's best not to rush into inductions. If your friends or family are impatient too and suggest you ask for an induction, you can explain about risks and choices, or show them this section of the book.

Let them know you'd prefer not to put yourself or your baby at risk unnecessarily. It's a shame their holiday ends a week earlier than your baby's birth, or that your baby might be born on Christmas day, but these things will pale into insignificance once you're holding a healthy baby in your arms, rather than looking at her through the perspex of a humidicrib.

> *'This is my first baby without induction. He's such a calm baby and I can't believe how much more in control I felt.'*
>
> **Helen, 26 years, third-time mum**

3

Can I bring on labour?

Having given my warning, there are a couple of natural techniques that may tip a woman into labour if she's ready. These are most likely to work if you've been having irregular (Braxton Hicks) contractions without going into proper labour.

• Many people believe having sex near your due date can help to send you into labour. Your man may worry that he will hurt the baby, but he won't. A man's semen contains prostaglandin, a hormone that helps to bring on labour (though it won't have much effect unless you're very close to going into labour already). During sex and climax, women release oxytocin, another hormone that induces labour.

• Nipple stimulation, which also releases oxytocin, can be as effective as sex in stimulating contractions. Tweak your nipples for a few minutes at a time. Feel silly? You can always do it in the bathroom, on your own – no one will know.

So, go ahead and have some fun producing oxytocin and prostaglandin! Otherwise, continue to wait. It's going to happen eventually, honest. Just remember, you won't have to go more than forty weeks and ten days without seeing your baby. And if your labour is not beginning, your baby is obviously very happy in there. Perhaps think of it as 'patience training', because you're going to need a lot of patience once your baby is born!

> *'I had to remind myself to sigh after each contraction – but it did make my shoulders relax.'*

Rae, 25 years, first-time mum

4

What happens with contractions?

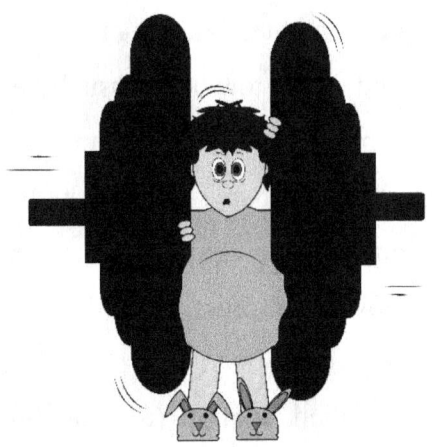

How does a contraction work? With each contraction, the bands of muscles within the womb tighten and pull the cervix upwards. As a result, your cervix begins to thin as it stretches. This process is referred to as effacement and is described as a percentage. So, if your cervix has not thinned at all, it's 0 per cent effaced; if it has thinned completely, it's one hundred percent percent effaced.

As labour continues, the contractions become stronger and closer together – usually every three to five minutes. Each contraction pushes downwards on the baby, causing the baby's head to put increasing pressure on the cervix. This constant downward pressure on the cervix causes it to open gradually and stay open. The opening process is called dilation (or dilatation) and is measured in centimetres. If dilation is 0 centimetres, your cervix is still closed; if it is ten centimetres, it is completely dilated – just the right size for your baby's head to pass through – and you will be ready to push.

Your labour is progressing if the baby is coming down lower (descent) or if the cervix is opening (dilation). So don't despair if you're not dilating quickly but the baby is coming down; it's all happening. As the bottom half of the womb gets thinner, the top muscles in the uterus become stronger and more powerful. The bigger, thicker muscle helps to push the baby down and through your pelvis in preparation for birth. This downward shift by the baby is called **descent**

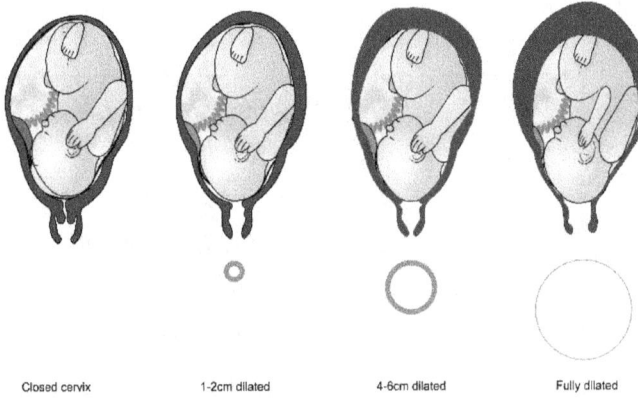

| Closed cervix | 1-2cm dilated | 4-6cm dilated | Fully dilated |

Cervix –thick-then thinning-then gone

Cervix-closed-slightly open-then fully open

For women having their first baby, it's common for descent to have occurred (i.e. for the baby to have 'dropped' into the pelvis) even before the first contraction or any sign of dilation. For women having their second baby, it is not uncommon for some dilation to occur before labour, even though the baby is still sitting quite high in the pelvis (not descending). Progress in labour is measured from the time you start regular contractions because these consistent contractions usually indicate good progress.

> *'When the midwife told me*
> *'You're five centimetres*
> *dilated,' I wanted to cry,*
> *Then she said, 'The first half*
> *is the slow part.' The rest*
> *certainly went quicker.'*
> **Tara, first time**

5

Will I be safe at home in early labour?

A resounding YES!

Think about animals. When an animal is preparing to birth, what does she do? She makes a nest or hides where she feels safe. The labour stops if the animal doesn't feel safe but starts again when she is comfortable in her surroundings.

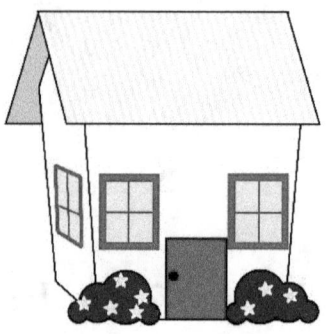

As humans, we make our nice nest at home where we feel safe. But when we go into early labour, our support people can tend to hurry us into the car and take us to hospital, a place that may make us nervous. If we are not in full labour, our labour could stop when we begin to feel nervous.

So, consider the option of waiting at home, where you feel safe and can shower or bath in privacy, rest, fiddle with baby clothes, or just chill out with your support people. If it really is the time, labour will progress and it won't slow down again or stop for a break.

Eventually, you will want to go to the hospital or birthing centre to feel safe, and that will be the right time for you to go.

Let's say it's 3 a.m. and you go to the toilet, as you do every night when your pregnant belly presses on your bladder. You notice you have some low-down, gripey, period-like pains that come and go. What should you do? I'd suggest going back to bed. If the pains aren't too bad, you don't even need to tell anyone. You can smile quietly in the darkness and wonder if this is it. If you wake up in the morning and the pains have gone, it's not time yet.

If the pains continue, rest is really important during the night. If the pains are twenty minutes apart, you will probably be able to doze for fifteen minutes between them. Make sure you do! The average length of labour for a first-time mum is fourteen to sixteen hours. (Of course, some labours are shorter and some are longer.)

So the more you rest now, the better you are going to handle those last few hours.

If it's the middle of the day, sit or stroll somewhere peaceful and do something to take your mind off the waiting. The more you try to hurry up your labour, the more it seems to slow down—frustrating, I know—but good to remember when people say they wish things would hurry up.

Tension and fear slow labour, and can make contractions more painful. If contractions have started to become painful and rest isn't an option, then you may feel like you want to move around. Vacuuming is great exercise; add some dance music and you'll swing into labour with all the right moves. Or maybe try some belly dancing – after all, you have a great belly!

Either way, be happy. It's happening. The world is a good place and sometime soon you're finally going to meet your baby. If your contractions are still very irregular, then rest is most important because you could be doing this for the next few days or even a week. Perhaps it's best not to wear your support people out by making them rub your back too early, or you'll miss them at the end when you really need them.

If the pains are regular, painful, and getting stronger and closer together, the birth is not so far away.

In early labour, your body begins to release endorphins (hormones that are the body's natural pain medication). Endorphins will be particularly helpful as your contractions increase in intensity, so it's important to get them flowing now by relaxing. You'll probably feel excited, and every now and then you might get the giggles. This is the smiley-face part of labour.

While you're in early labour, keep sipping water, eat if you feel like it, and go to the bathroom every two hours at least. There will come a time (in my experience, usually when your cervix is around two to four centimetres dilated) when you just won't feel happy at home any more, and you'll tell your support people that it's time to go. Listen to your body and you'll know.

If you do end up at the hospital a little early and the midwives give you the option to go home, take it. Even if you come back in half an hour, you'll have progressed your labour by relaxing a bit after dropping the strain that made you go to the hospital in the first place. Midwives won't care if you come back half a dozen times.

> *'My husband, Doug, was there for me. He was great when I got cranky. I couldn't have done it without him.'*
>
> **Noni, 23 years, first-time mum**

6

What if my waters haven't broken?

Some women's waters don't break until they start pushing, and some babies are even born inside the bag of amniotic fluid ('born in the caul'). In the old days, midwives used to say a caul baby would never drown. Sailors would buy the dried sac membranes from caul babies to take to sea to keep them safe. (Sorry, I'm getting off the track, but isn't it fascinating!)

Not so long ago, doctors and midwives often

used to break a mother's waters to make her labour progress faster, even if everything was happening normally. Nowadays, breaking the waters is usually done only to check the colour of the amniotic fluid if necessary, or to increase contractions for a reason. Otherwise, there's generally no need to interfere; a baby inside the sac is protected from infection and from complications arising from pressure on the umbilical cord, and you are protected from some of the discomfort of your baby's head pressing on the cervix.

If your waters need to be broken for a medical reason, a plastic instrument a bit like a crochet hook, or a long skinny instrument like a pair of tweezers, will be inserted into the vagina along the midwife or doctor's finger to catch and make a hole in the bottom of the sac. This lets the fluid out in gushes. There needs to be an opening in the cervix (i.e. some dilation) before the sac can be reached.

> *'At first, I thought she'd had too much lemonade. But the water kept coming, all over my new car-seat covers, and I started to panic that she'd have the baby there. We made it to the hospital.'*
>
> **Steve, 24 years, first-time**

7

What's the secret to breathing?

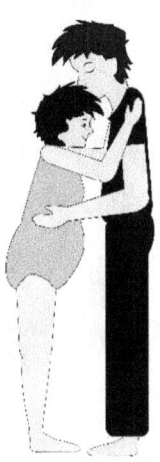

During birth, you have to breathe (you have no

choice!) The secret is to keep your breathing slow and steady. There's lot of books out there describing special ways to breathe in labour. If you want more detail, you should buy or borrow a book on breathing techniques, or find someone to go through it with you. Certain types of breathing can help more than others, but remember, you're training to manage the pain of birth, not to do a breathing exam.

Calmbirth® classes can be extremely helpful and are run all over Australia and New Zealand. If you have the time and money (it's often a personal class), Google 'calmbirth' to find your closest practitioner.

Practise breathing

You can practise breathing using this simple exercise:

Breathe in through your nose (as if your nostrils are going to stick together) while you push your belly out. Then breathe out through your mouth and let your belly sink towards your spine as you relax. Make up your own little ditty as you breathe, or use this to help you remember:

Breathe in through my nose,
push my belly to my clothes.

Breathe out through my mouth
and my belly goes south.

Breathing slowly and deeply like this takes

a bit of practice (it's probably not quite how you're used to breathing) but it helps to keep you calm. It works for me in lots of situations, including at the dentist! And these breaths are a good trick to have up your sleeve when it comes to pushing your baby out. Try to practise this breathing for a few minutes every day – perhaps just before you go to sleep.

You can also practise sighing at the beginning and end of a contraction. Sighing at the beginning of a contraction relaxes your pelvic floor muscles (try sighing and you'll be able to feel this happening). I believe this helps the cervix to stay relaxed and soft so that it can dilate more easily for birth. Sighing at the end of a contraction helps you let go of the tension you have picked up during the contraction. Anything that helps your body to a speedy and more comfortable birth is a good thing to practise. Try a slow sigh in and a slow sigh out: do you feel the weight of your body sink into the bed or chair? That's a good sigh and something else you could practise at night a few times before you go to sleep.

In labour

Once you're having contractions, remember the waves at the beach. At the beginning of a contraction (as you start to ride up one side of the wave), let out a sigh, and sigh again at the end (once you reach the bottom of the other side).

How you cope in the middle of the contraction (at the peak of the wave) depends on its intensity, but breathing as slowly and steadily as possible will help you to remained focussed.

Remember that it's all downhill from the peak of the wave. As you sigh at the end, try to go loose and floppy – relax your whole body. Feel the weight of your body sinking down. On average, in early labour, a contraction lasts about forty to sixty seconds, and the middle twenty to thirty seconds is hard work. The middle is often a good time to moan. (This sound can be disconcerting for your support person, but if you let them know that it helps during the contractions, they'll feel better and might even start doing it with you.)

Most women find that fixing their gaze on a single unmoving point – the window, the corner of the room or a quiet, motionless person – also helps them to stay focussed and remain calm.

> *Just staring at my partner's*
> *face kept me focused.*
>
> **Annie, three time mum**

8

Hospital and settling in

If you haven't already spoken to the hospital since your labour began, phone to tell them that you're coming. When you arrive, you and your birth partner might feel naturally anxious. Your contractions will probably be more painful by this stage and you'll have to walk into a place where you may not know anyone. Remember, it's okay. The midwives are there because they love this job and they're very good at it.

If you've called ahead, the midwives will have gone through your chart and birth plan. If you're lucky enough to have your own midwife who'll also be with you during labour, she'll be prepared to meet you at the hospital and will know everything you need and want. It's a great help if the midwife knows your birth plan because you might not be in the mood to explain your preferences. This cuts the time it takes for you to get into the shower or bath and start to feel more settled. Unpacking your things will also help to make you feel calmer.

Your body is a clever thing. Once you've settled in, more hormones will flood your bloodstream and suddenly you'll begin to feel tired. Majorly tired. I-don't-want-to-do-this-now-let's-do-it-tomorrow tired. Good! That's normal. That's your body helping you to stay relaxed and cope with the increasing intensity of the contractions. Believe it or not, you will learn to cope. Endorphins that started flowing because you stayed relaxed at home in early labour will now help you sail through contractions that you would have squirmed over a couple of hours ago. It's the endorphins that make you tired as they dull the intensity of the contractions and help you remain as loose as possible.

To release endorphins, you need dim lighting, quiet music (or no music if silence helps you concentrate), distant focus, calm people who are not chattering and distracting you, and trust in your caregiver.

Fear stops the release of endorphins (stopping natural pain relief) and produces adrenalin – the last thing you want when you're trying to relax during a contraction. So, don't let anyone you're not comfortable with into the birthing room. Let fear go and believe in your body; you're in a safe place and your body is designed to do just what it's doing.

Labouring

There are several things that can help to make your labour more comfortable.

Get off the bed

I'm not the only midwife who believes that lying on a bed is the most uncomfortable way to labour. Your baby has to descend through your pelvis, so lying down doesn't usually encourage a faster or more comfortable labour.

When you're lying down:

- the full weight of your baby will be pushing on your spine or hips, which is uncomfortable and makes it difficult for you to move

- your baby is more likely to become distressed, as blood flow decreases

- others in the room will be looking down on you, which can make it difficult for you to be assertive.

Standing or sitting upright, with the earth's gravity encouraging downward pressure and descent, is usually much more comfortable. Movement – rocking, swaying, and walking – also promotes progress and is less painful on your spine and hips. Some women are uncomfortable in any position except standing. No problem – hang on to those rails in the bathroom!

Use the bath/shower

Water is great for stimulating endorphins. Many women shake their head at the suggestion of a bath or shower but, in my experience, labour in water seems to progress much faster and with less pain than it does on a bed. Does faster and less painful sound good? Then give the water a try.

If you don't want a full shower or bath, try sitting on a birth ball (most hospitals have these – they look just like exercise balls) and ask your support person to run warm water over your belly – many women find this a huge relief.

The bath/shower has the following benefits:

- the warmth of the water offers pain relief and the sound is soothing

- in the shower, you can face the wall so that you are not distracted by anyone

- in the bath, you are surrounded by warmth and can float weightlessly while your body does its job.

Use a ball or a chair

Some women get great relief from leaning over a ball, beanbag or bed while someone rubs their back. Ask your support person to rub using an oil or cream to avoid raw skin.

Sitting on a ball or backwards on a chair with your support person behind you rubbing your back is often very helpful. Try using two pillows between you and the back of the chair (in front of you): one to bury your belly in and one to rest your forehead on.

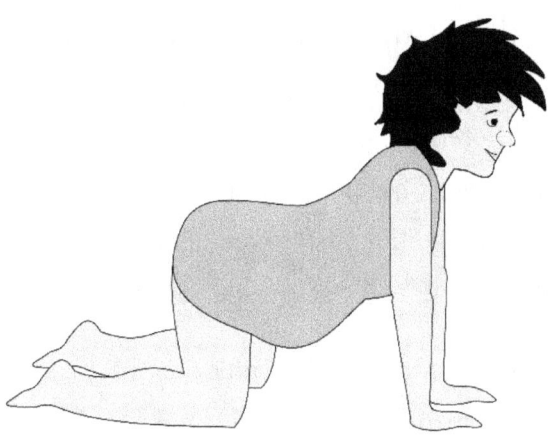

Breathe through the contractions as your support person rubs – it's very relaxing. Women often say they feel better with firm pressure during contractions and a softer massage, or no touch, in the break between. Practise this at home during your pregnancy. You can even give your partner a rub to see how they like it (but make sure that they do the bulk of the massaging, to build up their stamina!)

Use a heat pack

Heat packs and wheat bags are wonderful, too, but if you plan to use one, warn your support people beforehand. They will need to keep an eye on you because, during a strong contraction, boiling hot won't seem hot enough, and you're liable to scald yourself.

(We don't use hot water bottles in hospitals because women in strong labour unwrap them and put them straight on their skin for relief. I told you endorphins were strong!)

9

Checking on baby

For most women, pregnancy is a normal and natural life event. However, for some women, medical conditions and other risk factors mean extra monitoring is required to ensure both you and your baby remain as healthy as possible throughout pregnancy and labour. High-risk pregnancies can include multiple births and women with diabetes, heart problems or other medical conditions.

If you have some of these risk factors, you may need to give birth in one of the larger city hospitals, where you can be cared for by a specialist obstetrician and have access to services such as ultrasound and the neonatal intensive-care unit. If you live in the country and need this type of care, your local doctor or hospital may be able to share your care with the larger hospital and obstetrician, providing the opportunity for you to stay at home for most of your pregnancy and, if all goes well, during your labour as well.

But even healthy women at low risk can still expect a certain amount of monitoring and observation prior to the birth. On admission, a midwife will take your blood pressure, pulse and temperature, and will probably ask for a urine sample. She'll also want to get to know your baby through touch: she'll listen to the baby's heart rate and find out which position she is lying in. She'll ask when your contractions began and will time them. She'll also want to know the colour of any fluid you have lost/are losing.

Sometimes, the midwife or doctor might also

ask whether she can do a vaginal examination by feeling for the baby's head with her fingers. It's important to know exactly how dilated you are in labour if:

• you've asked for some medicated pain relief

• your labour seems to go on for longer than expected

• your baby's heart rate is slowing or accelerating more than expected.

Most hospitals no longer do a routine fetal-monitor trace of the baby's heart rate on arrival for low-risk women. However, if something crops up to increase your risk – for example, labour is too early, or you have a raised temperature, or your waters are broken and unusual fluid is draining – you'll be hooked up to a cardiotocograph monitor on admission. A CTG monitor is made up of two sensors that rest on your stomach. One is an ultrasound Doppler that 'hears' your baby's heartbeat and the other is a pressure gauge that 'feels' your contractions (the tightness of your belly when it hardens) pushing against it.

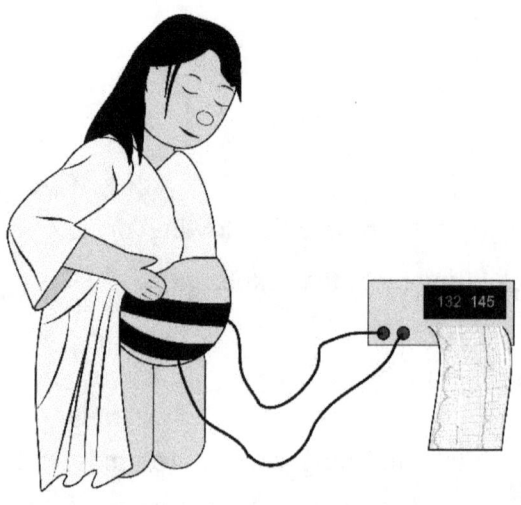

Cardiotocograph monitor

The CTG monitor produces a graph that is

divided into minutes, allowing the midwife or doctor to see how often your contractions come and how long they last. Because the baby's heart rate is recorded at the same time as your contractions, your carer can also see what the baby's heart response is to the contraction (for example, is your baby's heart rate slowing after contractions?). However, it's important to remember that CTGs are not infallible; sometimes, happy babies have suspicious CTG records, and vice versa.

It is appropriate for a CTG monitor to be used if:

- you already have some risk factors

- an intervention such as induction

is used

- something changes in your labour that could potentially affect your baby.

If everything is normal, the CTG monitor doesn't need to be used; in fact, because

it requires you to lie down, it has its own associated risks, such as:

- your pain may be felt more strongly,

  so you might need more medicated pain relief (see page 73)

- your labour might slow because you aren't able to move or stand up and make use of the help that gravity gives you

• without movement, the blood flow

to your womb and baby might lessen, making the baby unhappy and meaning that further monitoring is required.

Use of the CTG monitor should be weighed up against these extra risks because what was intended as a safety measure can affect how your labour progresses.

If the monitor isn't needed, it's still important to check that your baby's heart rate remains normal during labour; labour is hard work for both you and your baby, and the baby can get tired. Every fifteen to thirty minutes, your midwife will probably listen to the clop, clop of your baby's heart with a hand-held Doppler monitor after a contraction. This ensures that your baby is being monitored safely.

If you have no medical problems and your baby is well, remember that you have a choice in the type of monitoring you receive in labour, and it's okay to tell the midwife that you'd prefer the Doppler.

Sometimes everyone was too busy watching the machine to ask me how strong the contractions were.

Marie, mother of six

10

What if my labour needs to be induced?

If you're unwell – for example, if your blood pressure is up towards the end of pregnancy, or you have diabetes or a heart problem – then the risk of you and your baby becoming unwell may be more significant than the risks of intervention, and your doctor may decide to induce. In this case, the decision for induction is a medical one, rather than the fact that you might simply want your baby to be born before a particular date.

The good news is that if an induction is required, Mother Nature usually ensures that your body agrees and is ready with you. These inductions seem to be quicker and need less intervention than inductions carried out for non-medical reasons.

If your doctor tells you an induction is needed for medical reasons, here's what is most likely to happen. Before an induction is started, a fetal monitor (see page 59) will be strapped to your belly to make sure your baby's heart rate is healthy and your uterus doesn't become overstimulated. Then, one of two methods of medical induction will be used to produce a labour onset.

Prostaglandin

This method is as close to natural as possible, and is the most common at the moment. Prostaglandin gel will be inserted inside your vagina behind your cervix (it feels a bit like having a pap smear), or, alternatively, prostaglandin tape will be wrapped loosely around your cervix. The prostaglandin 'softens' your cervix and sends hormonal messages that tell your body it's time to go into labour. Afterwards, you'll need to stay still for about half an hour to help the prostaglandin absorb. You don't need to lie completely flat – just don't stand or move around too much. (In fact, it's best never to lie flat on your back with a pregnant belly because the weight of your uterus cuts down the blood flow to your baby by squashing the major blood vessels. You are likely to feel light-headed, too. If you tilt a little to one side – left is often better but not compulsory – then the light-headedness will disappear and your placenta will be able to work more efficiently.) While you're lying down, the fetal monitor will show the reaction your uterus has to these signals and how the baby's heart rate reacts to the onset of labour. A prostaglandin induction can take twenty-four or even forty-eight hours, and a couple of doses of prostaglandin.

Syntocinon

The other drug often used in medical induction is Syntocinon, an artificial form of the natural hormone oxytocin, which your body usually releases to start contractions.

Oxytocin is also naturally released after your baby is born, when you breastfeed, and helps slow the bleeding after birth by contracting the uterus.

Syntocinon is given through a drip into your veins. The fetal monitor will stay on for most or all of a Syntocinon induction, which is usually shorter and more intense than a prostaglandin induction. With Syntocinon, the contractions start slowly and get closer and more regular over a couple of hours of the drug being used. Often, if your cervix is dilated enough, your waters will be artificially broken when Syntocinon is given. This type of induced labour can be more intense than normal labour; you may need more pain relief to help you relax because the contractions come on more quickly (you may not have time to build up your endorphin levels like you do when labour starts naturally). But then, some women have fast and furious natural labours, too.

My labours are so fast we carry a cord clamp. We've never had to use it - but nearly.

Belle, mother of four

11

Drugs and pain relief

I saw your ears prick up at the mention of drugs. They are always available as back-up, so there's no need to be afraid of being in pain.

If your baby is facing the right way and you stay upright rather than lying on the bed, in most situations your endorphins will carry you to the end. But if the pain means you can't relax between contractions, or you become anxious and adrenalin kicks in, pain relief can allow you to doze for a couple of hours, regaining strength and control in order to push. And, in some circumstances, pain relief can even speed up labour.

The four most effective methods of pain relief during labour are:

1. Drugs you breathe in:

Gas (a mixture of nitrous oxide and oxygen, commonly called laughing gas) can be very useful, especially during the strong contractions prior to pushing. It reduces pain in two ways: it induces a feeling of pleasure (you'll need a good few breaths before you start to feel this, so don't give up); and the mental concentration required to suck the gas properly helps block out the sharpness of the strong contractions.

To use gas, breathe in and out through the mouthpiece or mask as the contraction builds. You are in control, and you can start and stop using it whenever you like.

Downside

Too much gas may make you and your baby sleepy. But the effect will wear off quite quickly once you stop breathing the gas.

2. Drugs injected into a muscle or under the skin

Morphine is a drug that mimics the way endorphins work. It lasts from two to four hours and can make you very sleepy (inclined to curl up on the bed). It can often bring on nausea and vomiting so is given with an anti-nausea drug.

If you find that your contractions are

becoming difficult to manage, morphine can help you to relax again.

Downsides

- If you're given morphine within an hour or so of birth (or in transition), the transfer of the drug from the placenta can make your baby quite sedated at birth and for a few hours afterwards. If you have morphine within four hours of giving birth, your baby will be observed for at least four hours afterwards to make sure that she is breathing well. Morphine can also affect early breastfeeding reflexes in your baby.

- If you don't like the feeling morphine gives you or it makes you very sick, there's not a lot you can do about it until it wears off.

3. Drugs injected into the spine

Spinal anaesthesia and epidural anaesthesia are great options if you're having a caesarean section or you are exhausted from a long labour. They numb your body from a certain level – your nipples or your waist – all the way to your feet, and you shouldn't feel pain, only pressure. (If someone pressed an ice cube against your body after this kind of anaesthesia, you'd feel the pressure but not the cold.)

A spinal anaesthetic is used mostly for caesarean births because it acts very quickly. A needle connected to a small tube is put into your back and the tube is fed into the sac that holds your spinal cord and fluid. The risk of headache afterwards is slightly greater with a spinal anaesthetic than with an epidural.

An epidural is used mostly to relieve pain during labour. It takes a little longer to act because the anaesthetic is injected into the space outside the sac. The tubing is left in until your baby is born so that more anaesthetic or narcotic can be injected as necessary. If you'd prefer to have an epidural early in your labour, it'd be a good idea to note this on your birth plan. Some hospitals promote epidurals more than others.

Downsides

- You'll need a drip in your arm in case your blood pressure falls.

- Because you don't have full sensation, it's often harder to push out your baby, and there's an increased risk of needing help (like forceps or a vacuum extraction) to ease your baby's head down the last bit of the birth canal. Watching with a mirror can help you push more effectively.

4. Subcutaneous water injections This method doesn't involve any drugs, but it can be really helpful for those who suffer severe back pain during labour. A tiny injection of sterile water is given just under the skin so that it blebs up in two to four places on your lower back. The injections are spread across a hand-sized area, over the painful part of your back. They are given during a contraction and while you are using gas, if possible, because they sting like the blazes. But they're usually worth it. I've seen women beside themselves with back pain (a pain score of ten out of ten) drop their score to a four within two minutes and to one or zero within five minutes. Subcutaneous water injections have no side effects for you or your baby, and they last for hours. Now that's a bargain! If you're interested in this option, check whether it is available at your hospital.

Downside

The injections sting for about thirty seconds when given.

> '*When I was deep in labour, I was so sleepy – I thought it couldn't be right, but it was the hormones kicking in. Being sleepy helped me breathe and relax between the pains.*'
>
> **Janet, mother of twins**

12

The stages of labour

Once you've reached three to four centimetres of dilation, you've begun the 'active' phase of labour, because the intense and regular contractions are strong enough to progressively open the cervix.

Strong labour

During most active labours, the contractions will be regular (every two–three minutes and lasting for at least one minute) and strong. You'll only get a minute or two of relief between contractions, so use this time well by dumping any tension with those outward sighs at the end of the contractions.

During contractions, drop your shoulders and close your eyes. Sink back and breathe slowly and deeply – in through your nose and out through your mouth, perhaps with a moan. Think about your baby and draw your breath right down into the base of your lungs. Imagine your breath activating the hormone receptors that will flood your body with more endorphins.

At this stage, the contractions are bringing the weight of your baby down onto your cervix, forcing it to open further and further. You will need your support people to speak in short sentences and quiet voices, and only about things that are to do with how they can help you. Are they rubbing in the right place? Too hard or soft? Do you need a sip of water? Do you need to go to the bathroom? (They should be reminding you to go at least every couple of hours.)

At the peak of each wave, imagine your cervix opening further (dilation). Your brain might suggest, 'I can't do this!' but your body is designed to do it, and is doing exactly what it should be. Believe it! Let go. Focus on getting through the next contraction, then forget it. Then focus on the next one.

It is important for your support people not to chatter in the background as you are trying to focus. (This is why you need to think about who you want in the room before labour begins) –It can be really useful to focus on a single point somewhere in the room and simply concentrate on breathing.

If you get to a stage where you feel your control start to slip, it's time to MOVE. Change position. Get out of the shower if that's where you are, and stomp around the room. Lean against people, walls, over a ball or bean bag and have someone rub your back. And when that gets crazy, MOVE again. Even if it's back into the shower. You're heading for transition. This is where your midwife and your support person should be the calm rocks in your ocean. This is where women amaze and inspire me. You are truly awesome.

Transition

Transition is the time when your body is forcing the last few centimetres of cervix out of the way of your baby's head. The pains will be quick, with little break in between – they might even double up so you get two pains together, then a little break, then a smaller pain and then a huge one. B*gger!

You might find yourself saying, 'I can't do this,' or

'I want to go home,' or 'It's all your fault, you b*stard!' to your partner.

(It's good to warn them beforehand that this might happen. Perhaps give them this book to read.) If you haven't had an epidural, you might start asking for one. However, epidurals take a little time to organise, perform and start to work. A drip has to be inserted beforehand, your blood pressure monitored and the necessary position for the procedure assumed – all while you are being buffeted by intense contractions.

It's a little tricky to achieve all these goals in the (usually) short time before you move from transition into the pushing stage, when the storm settles and you are back in control. It also becomes more difficult to push effectively with the lessened sensation. This is why the midwife or doctor might suggest that it's too late for an epidural.

You might wish the doctor could cut the baby out, right NOW! I see lots of women go through transition and I've been there myself. (Forgive your midwife if she's smiling; it's relief, because she knows you're almost there.) Hang in there. Keep breathing. At this stage you'll be very close to being able to push and do something with these powerful urges – you're on the home straight.

Pushing

Once your cervix has disappeared, you'll feel the urge to push. Usually, just before this urge begins, your contractions will settle down to every three or four minutes, giving you time to gather yourself. Often, nature will give you a breather of ten or more minutes without any contractions. A few women never seem to get the urge to push; in this case, wait a little longer and if it doesn't happen and the midwife tells you your cervix has disappeared, push anyway. This is where the breathing ditty can be very helpful.

I've spoken a few times about breathing and this is the time to really put it into practice. When the contraction starts, your womb has to do a heck of a lot of work, so help it by doing all of your pushing during the contraction, and ensure that you rest between contractions. You'll progress much faster if you're upright rather than on your back. Perhaps try sitting on the toilet – many women find this the most comfortable place.

Breathe in slowly and deeply through your nose, pushing your belly out, feeling the pressure in your stomach muscles; then breath out slowly and feel the pressure in your belly easing down into your bum as you do so.

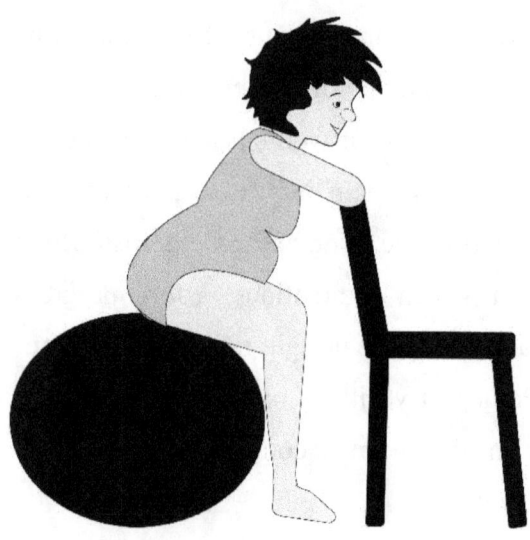

Remember, the secret to breathing is to keep it slow and steady. In my experience, a woman who breathes quietly in and out as her baby descends into the world remains calm and establishes a better oxygen flow for herself and her baby, resulting in an easier birth. The midwife will be with you all the time at this stage; she'll wait for you to feel the baby moving down and the start of the burning sensation as your vagina starts to stretch. Once she sees your baby's head, you'll need to decide where you want to have the baby – on the birth stool, standing, kneeling, on or beside the bed. Or, if you're in the bath or shower, you might like to remain there. When you can see the top of your baby's head and it doesn't go back between contractions, you're about to give birth. You might find yourself thinking, 'OMG, how?'

Remember, your body is designed to do this. Why do you think you have labia (the folds of skin outside the vagina)? All that extra skin is pulled outwards to expand the vaginal opening and allow the baby through. It will burn and sting, which is where warm water (a bath or even just a warm wet washer) will help. Try to push slowly. Try hard not to put your chin on your chest and shove that baby out of there because that's how tears can occur. (That's 'tear' as in rip, not 'tear' as in weep – though you might want to weep if it happens. Sometimes it happens anyway, especially if your baby is waving as she comes out! But most tears are minor.) Your vagina is designed to stretch slowly, to have a baby's head sit there while it stretches, and then to stretch more as the baby's head eases out. Your body is amazing!

It can be helpful to think about sighing your baby out rather than pushing. Remember, your strong contractions are pushing from above and a sigh will help to relax your pelvic floor muscles to let the baby birth. Many wise midwives say 'loose lips – loose perineum'! (The perineum is the plane of skin between the bottom of the vaginal opening and the anal opening, or anus.)

Once your baby's head is out, you've almost finished. Your baby is almost here. With the next contraction, her shoulders will come down. If her shoulders feel too tight to you, get on all fours with your bottom in the air and your knees together on your chest to provide the widest diameter for her to ease herself out.

> 'When she was near the end, she wanted me to take her home! And I couldn't do anything right. Lucky I'd been warned about transition. So it made me think we must be nearly there.'
>
> **Wally, 40 years, second-time dad**

13

The first hour after birth

The first few minutes after your baby is born are usually a blur. The contractions and the pushing are suddenly over, and your belly feels like a half-empty balloon, and your support team are crying. You look down to see your midwife or doctor lifting a slippery, tangled-limbed miniature person towards you as she wipes the goo off with a warm towel. Your baby will move and blink and start to flex her legs and arms, and you'll see that your baby is the most beautiful baby in the world, despite her squashed nose and mucky head.

If there's enough umbilical cord, she'll be lifted onto your chest, or, if the cord is short, onto your stomach. Someone will probably slip a needle into your thigh, if you have decided that's okay, containing a drug that helps the placenta to separate and lowers your risk of bleeding after birth, but you'll hardly notice because you'll be wrapping your arms around your baby and feeling how warm and precious she is and wondering how you created her. You are both awesome!

Recent studies suggest that a delay – even just a couple of minutes – in cutting the umbilical cord will allow your baby to keep more of the fetal blood from the placenta. This has many benefits, including increasing your baby's iron reserves. After this short delay, the midwife will hand the scissors to your birth partner or you to cut the cord, and your baby will be free. Congratulations!

Placenta delivery

Between five and thirty minutes later, you'll feel another contraction (you might glare at the midwife who told you it would all be over once the baby was born!) and then an urge to push. This push will evict the placenta (which has been keeping your baby alive during pregnancy). Midwives love placentas! Strange, I know, but this incredible disposable organ has been a heart–lung machine for your baby for a long time, and the bag that held the water and your baby is worth taking a look at. Truly. Not interested? Okay, just don't be surprised if the midwife asks whether you want a look.

If there's a long delay in the arrival of the placenta or if you're bleeding heavily before it is delivered (these situations are quite rare), your doctor may consider taking you to the operating theatre so that it can be removed under a general anaesthetic.

After the arrival of the placenta, someone will take your blood pressure and pulse, and feel around on your stomach for the now hard, grapefruit-sized uterus. They'll guide your hand to feel it, too. I know you want to play babies, but your midwife needs to have a feel because your incredible uterus needs to contract right down into itself to close off the blood vessels that were feeding the placenta. To help it contract, you'll be told to rub your uterus.

You will bleed a little after birth (use your maternity pads), but if you notice a constant trickle of blood or a pad full in an hour, the uterus is not doing its job and you need to tell the midwife.

If you managed to push slowly during the birth and didn't require stitches, your vagina will probably still feel a bit like a gravel truck just drove through, but in an hour or so, you'll be able to have a shower, which will help hugely. Your baby is amazing. You are amazing.

If you do require stitches, the area will be numbed with local anaesthetic. After several days, the stitches fall out – they don't need to be removed. A cool compress on your bottom helps with any swelling.

Welcome!

And now, a huge welcome to your little one. You're a mother. OMG.

Let's think about your baby. For nine months, she's been buoyantly suspended in a warm bath, with muted sounds and swaying movements her only contact with the outside world. But over the last few hours, she's been pushed this way and that until, finally, she's squashed then ejected into a bright, noisy, cold world – huge changes.

After having all her needs fulfilled inside you, she suddenly has to look after herself by breathing, crying and moving.

The one stable thing in her world is you, her mother. Her skin is pressed to yours, her nose buried in your skin – which she needs to smell and identify as yours – and her hands and knees knead your body as she wriggles in distress. You murmur to her, hold her to you, and she hears your voice – the voice she's heard through a watery filter for as long as she can remember – and she stops, listens and finally begins to relax.

Skin-to-skin

This is not the time to hand your baby to your mother-in-law or even the baby's father, unless you're not well. Right now, no one needs to know the exact weight of your baby, to immunise her or try clothes on her. She needs skin-to-skin contact with you for at least one hour after birth to acclimatise to this new world. You are the single most important factor in her life at this moment. If, for some reason, you can't hold her, then she needs another person to hold her, preferably skin-to-skin. I have no problem asking a man to put his sticky baby inside his shirt for an hour until mum can take over. I've done it with sisters and nanas, too. Nobody complains.

The great thing about-skin-to skin contact is that your baby stays warm and feels safe. For years, midwives used to wrap babies up in blankets for hours to warm them; where possible, this practice has been replaced by skin-to-skin contact that warms them like toast in as little as half an hour.

Lovely for mum, lovely for baby.

Surroundings

There are a couple of other things you can do to make your baby's world more comfortable in her first twenty-four hours.

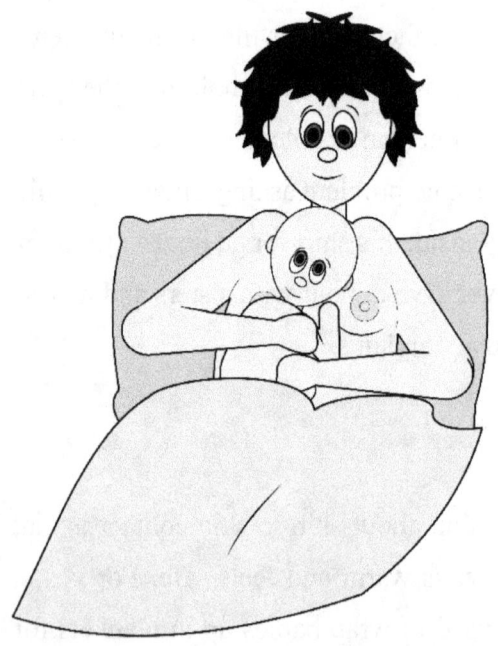

During this time, your baby is almost painfully sensitive to strong perfumes, because she is most interested in smelling (as well as looking at, listening to and tasting) you.

When you have your shower after the birth, try not to wash all the amniotic fluid scent from your breasts, and don't use scented body wash, shampoo or even deodorant in your baby's first twenty-four hours. We don't usually bath your baby during this time, either.

Your baby's sensitivity to smells and her likely confusion in the first twenty-four hours is something to share with your visitors before your baby is born. (You can imagine what happens

if a visitor wearing strong perfume holds your new baby against their neck – eww!)

In a perfect world, you could enforce the 'no one except Mum and Dad' cuddle rule for twenty-four hours – your baby would thank you for it. In reality, it can be a little difficult, but people with babies of their own are usually very understanding. With the others, you could ask them to read this section of the book if they have trouble understanding.

Try to keep the room dim and peaceful; this will encourage your baby to feel comfortable enough to look for a feed.

Julie wasn't well enough to have him on her chest so they made me take my shirt off. Our son was all sticky but it was the most amazing thing when he snuggled in and stopped crying. They threw a blanket over both of us. He didn't get cold like our first son did.'

Colin, 41 years,

second-time dad

14

Breastfeeding

Some babies seem to be born knowing how to breastfeed, some benefit from a little guidance, and for some mums, the stars don't align easily. If you go into labour assuming you'll breastfeed, you're more likely to do so, but I've also learnt how important it is to let your baby find her way by herself for the first feed. So, let's talk about cues and steps that can help your baby find her way more easily.

Your baby's first feed

In her first hour, your baby will look, listen, smell and taste you. And she'll yearn for your touch. Gently stroking her back in one direction as she lies against your skin will soothe her and not interfere with her search for the breast. Her lips should be lovely and pink – if they're not, check with your midwife, especially if you've had some morphine during labour.

Imagine that it's about ten minutes after birth. Your baby's in the hollow between your breasts. Your hands are gently stroking down her back, and she's sniffing the amniotic fluid, which is so familiar to her, on your skin. Her little feet have started to gently rub up and down against your tummy under the blanket that covers you both. The feel of her feet on your tummy makes your body release hormones to control bleeding, as well as encouraging colostrum (your protein-rich first milk) to flow in your breast.

Now she's gazing up at you and her pupils are huge as her eyes begin to circle your face. This circling is called 'tracking'. She's learning to recognise the way you look. The sound of your voice when you talk to her reinforces the fact that her mother's voice belongs to this face.

Gradually, she begins to put her hands to her mouth and she may dribble a little saliva onto her fingers. She begins to search your skin and breasts with her tiny wet fingers or little bunched fists. Your body makes more hormones in response to this touch so that the colostrum will be there when she's ready to feed. She starts to move her head from side to side and towards your breasts. Her hand goes to her mouth again, and perhaps her chin touches your breast a few times.

Next, her head begins to bob up and down as she stretches her neck and decides where she's aiming – until, suddenly, she jerks herself onto the chosen breast. She achieves this all by herself under your hands! Can you imagine that? Babies are amazing.

Now her face is against your skin and she's bobbing up and down. When she's happy with where she is, she sinks her chin into your breast again and her tongue starts to search out the areola (the darker brown circle around your nipple) and your nipple.

Letting your baby lick you and stretch her tongue is very important – this is where many of us come unstuck. Your baby needs to learn to push her tongue forward before she feeds. If she's pushed onto the breast by someone before she's learnt to stretch her tongue out, there's an increased risk that she'll damage your nipple later by keeping her tongue back; this is where a pain cycle – which often results in women giving up on breastfeeding – can start. So, let her find her way. Don't rush her. Remember, your baby is learning her first really important skill.

If you're worried about this, I suggest including in your birth plan the fact that you'd like your baby to find her first feed for herself, without help. Ask your partner to back you up on this in case someone forgets and tries to help your baby onto your breast.

When she does start to feed, allow your baby to do it her way. If her sucking stings or feels sharply uncomfortable, slip a finger into the corner of her mouth to break the suction and let her try again. Simply allowing these few steps to happen naturally and slowly can have a great impact on your entire breastfeeding experience.

Continuing to breastfeed

After that first feed, ask for as much help as you need from the midwives and the lactation consultant, when she's available. And don't be afraid to ask; they really want breastfeeding to be a special and rewarding time for both you and your baby.

Once you're home, try to surround yourself with supportive friends, especially those who are also breastfeeding; this will boost your confidence. The Australian Breastfeeding Association has a helpful website (www. breastfeeding.asn.au) full of contacts and resources. Don't be afraid to use them.

And remember that love doesn't come from the breast, so if you're unable to breastfeed, for whatever reason, please don't torment yourself over it; these tips might help to give you a better chance next time.

Breastfeeding took baby and I a while to figure out but I'm so glad we kept at it. I love it now.

Bianca,

first time mum

15

Making the most of your hospital stay

If you and your baby are well, it's your choice how long you stay in hospital – anywhere from four hours to a few days, depending on your hospital or birthing centre, and whether you have healthcare cover. Make the most of your time there. Before you leave, make sure the midwives have answered your questions on how to:

- breastfeed (you might like to try a few different techniques)

- express milk

- change nappies

- bath your baby (and check the umbilical cord)

- wrap your baby for sleeping.

Also, ask a midwife to go over the history of your labour with you: how long it lasted and any variations from normal. (Once you're home, it's much harder to access this information.) Knowing exactly what happened is likely to help you in future births. If anything happened that you want to avoid next time, or something didn't happen that you would have liked, make a note of it and put it in your next birth plan. By now you'll understand why it's important to make birth the most positive experience possible. Maybe begin your next birth plan now, while things are fresh in your mind.

'We wrote down that I'd like to cut the cord, and that I'd like to lift our son David onto Judy's chest after he was born. I don't think

I would have remembered at the time, but our midwife made sure it happened.'

**Pete, 28 years,
first-time dad**

16

Your birth plan

You know by now that birth is not a show you have to perform solo. You're the team leader; your birth partner (this could be your man, your mum, your best friend, your sister or whoever you choose) is your major advocate; and your extra support people are the infrastructure. Your midwife will be there for you and your baby in labour, consulting with your doctor when needed.

Everyone on your birth team should know their

stuff and be there for you – not you for them. When designing a birth plan, talk with them about what you would like to happen (and perhaps suggest that they read this book after you). A birth plan is the best way to remind your team of what you would prefer to happen at your baby's birth.

Your birth plan needs to be written down so that things aren't forgotten during the excitement of the birth. However, the plan is not set in stone; it can change if necessary, to ensure a well baby and a well mother.

Here are some examples of the sorts of notes people write in their birth plans:

• I want only my partner and my mum in the room when I'm giving birth. (This is a great one if you have a persistent friend or relative who's hard to say no to. The midwife won't have any trouble keeping them out.)

• If I'm less than three centimetres dilated when

I come in to hospital, I want to go home again. (Staying in hospital before active labour increases the risk of unnecessary interventions.)

• If my waters break and I don't start contractions, I'd like to wait at least twenty-four (if I have no risk factors) before my labour is aided by drugs.

• If I have no risk factors, I would prefer not to have an admission CTG but to have my baby monitored by the midwife using a Doppler.

- During my labour, I wish to spend as little time as possible lying on the bed.

- I wish to use the shower and bath for pain relief before I consider medicated relief.

- I'd like to give birth in an upright position.

- I wish to have uninterrupted skin-to-skin contact with my baby for at least one hour after birth, and breastfeed before I leave the birthing suite.

- I want to just go with the flow, take it as it comes. (If you don't want to plan.)

- I want a photo with my baby but no 'down below' shots. (One of my favourite mementos of birth is a photo that's angled so it catches mum, dad, baby and the clock on the wall as soon as possible after birth. I love looking to see how old – in minutes – baby was when the photo was taken.)

These are just ideas. You could have one thing on your birth plan or you could have ten. Give a copy of your birth plan to your midwife for your notes and pack another copy in your hospital bag so that you always have it with you.

'I have to have my own pillow and doona.

*And my music. It makes me feel
safe.*

*Then I can
relax.'*

**Gail, 31 years, second-time
mum**

17

Your hospital bag

Pack a bag for the hospital early – you don't want to be trying to pack after your contractions have started. Don't take too much (you might not have much storage space in hospital) but do take anything that you think might make your labour more comfortable. Check what the hospital supplies and what it doesn't. Here is a list of what I think are the basics:

- A copy of your birth plan

- A sarong or big T-shirt that you can walk

around in. Make sure that it's comfortable and easy for the midwife to lift to check your baby's heart rate. If you're shy about your breasts, you could also pack a stretchy crop top or the top half of your swimmers (good in the shower).

• Dressing gown and slip-on footwear

• A shower cap to keep your hair dry and a hair band to keep it out of your face

• Soap on a rope or shower gel, so that the person rubbing your back in the shower doesn't keep losing the tiny hospital soap

• Toiletries

- If you like, your favourite music, because it transports you and makes you feel like the powerful person you are. (Most birthing suites have a CD player, but it's worth checking; if they don't, pack an iPod.)

- An unscented oil for massage when not in the shower (scented oils can become too heavy in a closed room)

- Socks – your feet can get cold in labour!

- Your own pillow if you love it, because neck cricks are the last thing you need

- A heat pack or wheat bag

- Disposable underpants – enjoy the glorious luxury of throwing out undies you don't want to wash

- Maternity pads

- Enough food and drinks to keep the support people going so that they don't have to leave to get supplies. Take some refreshments for yourself, too, but in my experience, a woman in strong labour is rarely interested in food. (All you will probably want is water to sip – and ice can be soothing, so make sure your support person finds the ice machine on the ward.)

- Camera and spare batteries

- A list of phone numbers of those you want to ring after the birth, and enough credit or change if you have to ring from a public phone

- Clothes (including a hat), nappies

  (check whether these are supplied by the hospital) and a bunny rug/muslin square for your new baby

- Knowledge, awareness and confidence

'Our midwife explained why some things had to change because our baby became tired during labour. We were okay with that when we understood why.'

Simon, 34 years, second-time dad

18

A quick word on the unexpected

As a labouring woman, you're not sick; you're simply completing a normal healthy process called childbirth. Sometimes, unexpected events occur or risks are present that require intervention. That's why we don't usually have our babies alone, without backup.

If something unusual happens to you or your baby during labour (or any other time) and you feel scared, ask questions, talk to your midwife or doctor and tell your team how you're feeling. Communication is hugely important at this time.

You are about to embark on an amazing journey. Prepare yourself with knowledge and awareness of the choices available. Have faith in your team. And, most importantly, have faith in yourself and your instincts because you are truly amazing.

Warmest wishes for you and your baby.

Fiona

Acknowledgements

With thanks to Annie Seaton who encouraged me to publish this second edition and assisting me with the work to make it e-accessible.

To Bettina Dwyer for the illustrations.

To Rae Condon, midwife and friend, whose calm, belief and good sense reminds me of what a midwife is.

And to my darling husband, Ian, my own rock and hero, my support person in labour and my best friend.

And most of all, my sincerest gratitude to all the awesome mothers whose births I've had the privilege of sharing over the last thirty years.

Thank you.

www.ingramcontent.com/pod-product-compliance
Lightning Source LLC
Chambersburg PA
CBHW060348190526
45169CB00002B/520